GUT HEALTH COOKBOOK FOR WOMEN

A Delicious and Holistic Cookbook to Support Women's Health

Dr Lily Morgan

COPYRIGHT PAGE

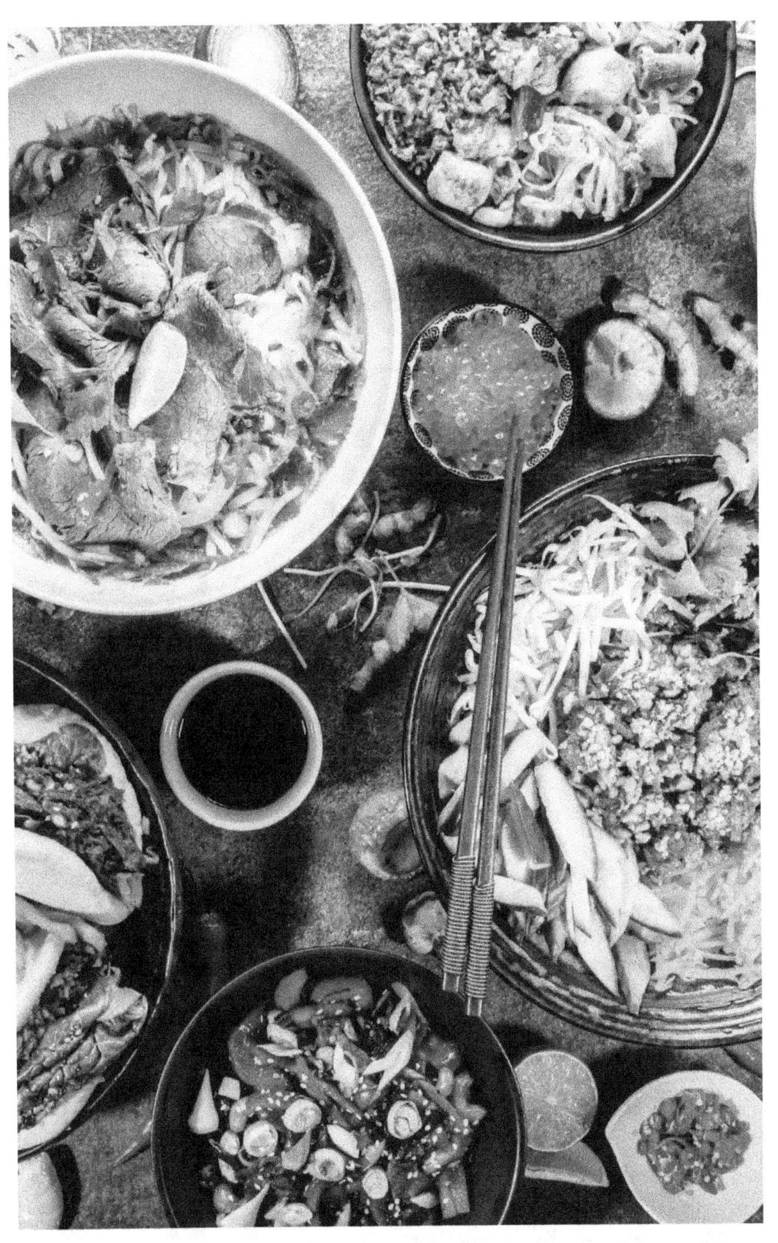

TABLE OF CONTENTS

Chapter 3: Lunch Recipes 39

Chapter 6: Desserts 88

INTRODUCTION

I n today's fast-paced world, maintaining good health is of paramount importance, especially for women. One aspect of health that has gained significant attention in recent years is gut health. The gut, often referred to as the "second brain," plays a crucial role in overall well-being, influencing everything from digestion to immune function and even mental health. This chapter serves as an essential foundation for understanding the significance of gut health and its specific relevance to women.

Understanding Gut Health and Its Importance

In this section, we delve into the intricacies of gut health and its vital role in maintaining overall wellness. We explore the gastrointestinal system's functions, emphasizing how it acts as a complex ecosystem populated by trillions of microorganisms, collectively known as the gut microbiota. We examine the delicate balance between beneficial and harmful bacteria and its impact on digestion, nutrient absorption, and the immune system.

How Gut Health Affects Women's Well-being

This section focuses on the unique ways gut health influences women's overall well-being. We explore the intricate connection between gut health and hormonal balance, particularly during various life stages such as menstruation, pregnancy, and menopause. Additionally, we discuss the role of gut health in managing conditions specific to women, including polycystic ovary syndrome (PCOS), endometriosis, and vaginal health.

Tips for Improving Gut Health

Here, we provide practical and actionable tips for improving gut health. We delve into dietary modifications, emphasizing the importance of a diverse and balanced diet rich in fiber, prebiotics, and probiotics. We also discuss the significance of stress management, regular exercise, and adequate sleep in promoting a healthy gut. Furthermore, we explore the potential benefits of certain supplements and explore strategies for reducing the intake of gut-damaging substances like alcohol and processed foods.

Essential Ingredients for a Gut-Healthy Diet

This section delves into the key ingredients that support gut health. We highlight various foods that are rich in probiotics, such as fermented vegetables, yogurt, and kefir. Furthermore, we emphasize the importance of prebiotic-rich foods, including whole grains, onions, garlic, and bananas, in nourishing the beneficial gut bacteria. Additionally, we explore the benefits of consuming fiber-rich foods, omega-3 fatty acids, and antioxidant-packed fruits and vegetables.

Tools and Equipment for Cooking Gut-Healthy Meals

In this final section, we provide an overview of the essential tools and equipment necessary for preparing gut-healthy meals. We discuss the importance of investing in high-quality cookware, such as stainless steel or cast-iron pans, to minimize exposure to harmful chemicals. Furthermore, we explore the benefits of using kitchen appliances like blenders, food processors, and slow cookers to create gut-friendly recipes with ease. Additionally, we offer tips on meal planning, food storage, and batch cooking to support a gut-healthy lifestyle.

Chapter 1: 30 Day Meal Plan

Week 1:

Day 1:

Breakfast: Gut-Healing Overnight Chia Pudding

Lunch: Gut-Healing Chicken and Vegetable Stir-Fry

Dinner: Gut-Friendly Grilled Salmon with Lemon and Dill

Snack: Gut-Healing Turmeric Hummus with Veggie Sticks

Dessert: Gut-Healing Mixed Berry Parfait with Coconut Yogurt

Smoothie: Gut-Healing Green Detox Smoothie

Day 2:

Breakfast: Energizing Quinoa Breakfast Bowl

Lunch: Quinoa Salad with Roasted Vegetables

Dinner: Gut-Soothing Roasted Chicken with Herbs

Snack: Gut-Nourishing Greek Yogurt Parfait with Berries

Dessert: Gut-Nourishing Dark Chocolate Avocado Mousse

Smoothie: Gut-Nourishing Berry Blast Smoothie

Day 3:

Breakfast: Turmeric Ginger Smoothie Bowl

Lunch: Gut-Nourishing Greek Salad

Dinner: Gut-Nourishing Quinoa-Stuffed Bell Peppers

Snack: Gut-Friendly Guacamole with Baked Tortilla Chips

Dessert: Gut-Friendly Banana and Walnut Bread

Smoothie: Gut-Friendly Mango and Spinach Smoothie

Day 4:

Breakfast: Gut-Nourishing Avocado Toast

Lunch: Gut-Friendly Lentil Soup

Dinner: Gut-Healing Shrimp and Vegetable Stir-Fry

Snack: Gut-Soothing Cucumber and Tzatziki Bites

Dessert: Gut-Soothing Chia Seed Pudding with Mango

Smoothie: Gut-Soothing Papaya and Pineapple Smoothie

Day 5:

Breakfast: Berry and Kale Breakfast Smoothie

Lunch: Mediterranean Chickpea Salad

Dinner: Gut-Friendly Lentil Curry

Snack: Gut-Healthy Almond and Date Energy Balls

Dessert: Gut-Healthy Blueberry Oat Bars

Smoothie: Gut-Healthy Chocolate Banana Smoothie

Day 6:

Breakfast: Gut-Friendly Vegetable Omelet

Lunch: Gut-Soothing Salmon and Asparagus Parcels

Dinner: Gut-Soothing Sweet Potato and Chickpea Curry

Snack: Gut-Nourishing Roasted Beetroot and Goat Cheese Crostini

Dessert: Gut-Nourishing Coconut Milk Rice Pudding

Smoothie: Gut-Nourishing Matcha Green Tea Smoothie

Day 7:

Breakfast: Buckwheat Pancakes with Blueberry Compote

Lunch: Gut-Healthy Turkey and Vegetable Wrap

Dinner: Gut-Healthy Turkey Meatballs with Zucchini Noodles

Snack: Gut-Healing Kale Chips

Dessert: Gut-Healing Baked Apples with Cinnamon and Almonds

Smoothie: Gut-Healing Turmeric and Ginger Smoothie

Week 2:

Day 8:

Breakfast: Spinach and Mushroom Frittata

Lunch: Spinach and Feta Stuffed Bell Peppers

Dinner: Gut-Nourishing Baked Cod with Garlic and Herbs

Snack: Gut-Friendly Zucchini Fritters

Dessert: Gut-Friendly Raspberry Coconut Ice Cream

Smoothie: Gut-Friendly Avocado and Kale Smoothie

Day 9:

Breakfast: Gut-Soothing Acai Bowl

Lunch: Gut-Healing Sweet Potato and Black Bean Burrito Bowl

Dinner: Gut-Healing Stuffed Cabbage Rolls

Snack: Gut-Soothing Roasted Chickpeas with Spices

Dessert: Gut-Soothing Pumpkin Spice Energy Bites

Smoothie: Gut-Soothing Blueberry and Almond Butter Smoothie

Day 10:

Breakfast: Cinnamon Apple Quinoa Porridge

Lunch: Butternut Squash and Quinoa Stuffed Portobello Mushrooms

Dinner: Gut-Friendly Vegetarian Chili

Snack: Gut-Healthy Smoked Salmon Cucumber Roll-Ups

Dessert: Gut-Healthy Chocolate Chip Zucchini Bread

Smoothie: Gut-Healthy Watermelon and Mint Smoothie

Day 11:

Breakfast: Zucchini and Sweet Potato Breakfast Hash

Lunch: Gut-Nourishing Cauliflower Rice Sushi Rolls

Dinner: Gut-Soothing Moroccan Vegetable Tagine

Snack: Gut-Nourishing Stuffed Mushrooms with Spinach and Feta

Dessert: Gut-Nourishing Strawberry Chia Jam Thumbprint Cookies

Smoothie: Gut-Nourishing Peach and Coconut Smoothie

Day 12:

Breakfast: Gut-Healing Overnight Chia Pudding

Lunch: Gut-Healing Chicken and Vegetable Stir-Fry

Dinner: Gut-Friendly Grilled Salmon with Lemon and Dill

Snack: Gut-Healing Turmeric Hummus with Veggie Sticks

Dessert: Gut-Healing Mixed Berry Parfait with Coconut Yogurt

Smoothie: Gut-Healing Green Detox Smoothie

Day 13:

Breakfast: Energizing Quinoa Breakfast Bowl

Lunch: Quinoa Salad with Roasted Vegetables

Dinner: Gut-Soothing Roasted Chicken with Herbs

Snack: Gut-Nourishing Greek Yogurt Parfait with Berries

Dessert: Gut-Nourishing Dark Chocolate Avocado Mousse

Smoothie: Gut-Nourishing Berry Blast Smoothie

Day 14:

Breakfast: Turmeric Ginger Smoothie Bowl

Lunch: Gut-Nourishing Greek Salad

Dinner: Gut-Nourishing Quinoa-Stuffed Bell Peppers

Snack: Gut-Friendly Guacamole with Baked Tortilla Chips

Dessert: Gut-Friendly Banana and Walnut Bread

Smoothie: Gut-Friendly Mango and Spinach Smoothie

Week 3:

Day 15:

Breakfast: Gut-Nourishing Avocado Toast

Lunch: Gut-Friendly Lentil Soup

Dinner: Gut-Healing Shrimp and Vegetable Stir-Fry

Snack: Gut-Soothing Cucumber and Tzatziki Bites

Dessert: Gut-Soothing Chia Seed Pudding with Mango

Smoothie: Gut-Soothing Papaya and Pineapple Smoothie

Day 16:

Breakfast: Berry and Kale Breakfast Smoothie

Lunch: Mediterranean Chickpea Salad

Dinner: Gut-Friendly Lentil Curry

Snack: Gut-Healthy Almond and Date Energy Balls

Dessert: Gut-Healthy Blueberry Oat Bars

Smoothie: Gut-Healthy Chocolate Banana Smoothie

Day 17:

Breakfast: Gut-Friendly Vegetable Omelet

Lunch: Gut-Soothing Salmon and Asparagus Parcels

Dinner: Gut-Soothing Sweet Potato and Chickpea Curry

Snack: Gut-Nourishing Roasted Beetroot and Goat Cheese Crostini

Dessert: Gut-Nourishing Coconut Milk Rice Pudding

Smoothie: Gut-Nourishing Matcha Green Tea Smoothie

Day 18:

Breakfast: Buckwheat Pancakes with Blueberry Compote

Lunch: Gut-Healthy Turkey and Vegetable Wrap

Dinner: Gut-Healthy Turkey Meatballs with Zucchini Noodles

Snack: Gut-Healing Kale Chips

Dessert: Gut-Healing Baked Apples with Cinnamon and Almonds

Smoothie: Gut-Healing Turmeric and Ginger Smoothie

Day 19:

Breakfast: Spinach and Mushroom Frittata

Lunch: Spinach and Feta Stuffed Bell Peppers

Dinner: Gut-Nourishing Baked Cod with Garlic and Herbs

Snack: Gut-Friendly Zucchini Fritters

Dessert: Gut-Friendly Raspberry Coconut Ice Cream

Smoothie: Gut-Friendly Avocado and Kale Smoothie

Day 20:

Breakfast: Gut-Soothing Acai Bowl

Lunch: Gut-Healing Sweet Potato and Black Bean Burrito Bowl

Dinner: Gut-Healing Stuffed Cabbage Rolls

Snack: Gut-Soothing Roasted Chickpeas with Spices

Dessert: Gut-Soothing Pumpkin Spice Energy Bites

Smoothie: Gut-Soothing Blueberry and Almond Butter
Smoothie

Day 21:

Breakfast: Cinnamon Apple Quinoa Porridge

Lunch: Butternut Squash and Quinoa Stuffed Portobello
Mushrooms

Dinner: Gut-Friendly Vegetarian Chili

Snack: Gut-Healthy Smoked Salmon Cucumber Roll-Ups

Dessert: Gut-Healthy Chocolate Chip Zucchini Bread

Smoothie: Gut-Healthy Watermelon and Mint Smoothie

Week 4:

Day 22:

Breakfast: Zucchini and Sweet Potato Breakfast Hash

Lunch: Gut-Nourishing Cauliflower Rice Sushi Rolls

Dinner: Gut-Soothing Moroccan Vegetable Tagine

Snack: Gut-Nourishing Stuffed Mushrooms with Spinach
and Feta

Dessert: Gut-Nourishing Strawberry Chia Jam Thumbprint
Cookies

Smoothie: Gut-Nourishing Peach and Coconut Smoothie

Day 23:

Breakfast: Gut-Healing Overnight Chia Pudding

Lunch: Gut-Healing Chicken and Vegetable Stir-Fry

Dinner: Gut-Friendly Grilled Salmon with Lemon and Dill

Snack: Gut-Healing Turmeric Hummus with Veggie Sticks

Dessert: Gut-Healing Mixed Berry Parfait with Coconut
Yogurt

Smoothie: Gut-Healing Green Detox Smoothie

Day 24:

Breakfast: Energizing Quinoa Breakfast Bowl

Lunch: Quinoa Salad with Roasted Vegetables

Dinner: Gut-Soothing Roasted Chicken with Herbs

Snack: Gut-Nourishing Greek Yogurt Parfait with Berries

Dessert: Gut-Nourishing Dark Chocolate Avocado Mousse

Smoothie: Gut-Nourishing Berry Blast Smoothie

Day 25:

Breakfast: Turmeric Ginger Smoothie Bowl

Lunch: Gut-Nourishing Greek Salad

Dinner: Gut-Nourishing Quinoa-Stuffed Bell Peppers

Snack: Gut-Friendly Guacamole with Baked Tortilla Chips

Dessert: Gut-Friendly Banana and Walnut Bread

Smoothie: Gut-Friendly Mango and Spinach Smoothie

Day 26:

Breakfast: Berry and Kale Breakfast Smoothie

Lunch: Mediterranean Chickpea Salad

Dinner: Gut-Friendly Lentil Curry

Snack: Gut-Healthy Almond and Date Energy Balls

Dessert: Gut-Healthy Blueberry Oat Bars

Smoothie: Gut-Healthy Chocolate Banana Smoothie

Day 27:

Breakfast: Gut-Friendly Vegetable Omelet

Lunch: Gut-Soothing Salmon and Asparagus Parcels

Dinner: Gut-Soothing Sweet Potato and Chickpea Curry

Snack: Gut-Nourishing Roasted Beetroot and Goat Cheese Crostini

Dessert: Gut-Nourishing Coconut Milk Rice Pudding

Smoothie: Gut-Nourishing Matcha Green Tea Smoothie

Day 28:

Breakfast: Buckwheat Pancakes with Blueberry Compote

Lunch: Gut-Healthy Turkey and Vegetable Wrap

Dinner: Gut-Healthy Turkey Meatballs with Zucchini Noodles

Snack: Gut-Healing Kale Chips

Dessert: Gut-Healing Baked Apples with Cinnamon and Almonds

Smoothie: Gut-Healing Turmeric and Ginger Smoothie

Day 29:

Breakfast: Spinach and Mushroom Frittata

Lunch: Spinach and Feta Stuffed Bell Peppers

Dinner: Gut-Nourishing Baked Cod with Garlic and Herbs

Snack: Gut-Friendly Zucchini Fritters

Dessert: Gut-Friendly Raspberry Coconut Ice Cream

Smoothie: Gut-Friendly Avocado and Kale Smoothie

Day 30:

Breakfast: Gut-Soothing Acai Bowl

Lunch: Gut-Healing Sweet Potato and Black Bean Burrito Bowl

Dinner: Gut-Healing Stuffed Cabbage Rolls

Snack: Gut-Soothing Roasted Chickpeas with Spices

Dessert: Gut-Soothing Pumpkin Spice Energy Bites

Smoothie: Gut-Soothing Blueberry and Almond Butter Smoothie

Congratulations on completing the 30-day meal plan! You've nourished your gut health with a variety of delicious and nutritious recipes. Remember to continue practicing a healthy and balanced diet to support your well-being.

Chapter 2: Breakfast Recipes

In this chapter, we will explore ten delicious and nourishing breakfast recipes that promote gut health. These recipes are designed to kick-start your day with a burst of flavor and provide the necessary nutrients to support your digestive system.

Gut-Healing Overnight Chia Pudding

Ingredients:

- 1/4 cup chia seeds
- 1 cup almond milk (or any non-dairy milk)
- 1 tablespoon pure maple syrup
- 1/2 teaspoon vanilla extract
- Fresh berries, for topping
- Chopped nuts, for topping

Instructions:

1. In a bowl, combine the chia seeds, almond milk, maple syrup, and vanilla extract. Stir well to combine.

2. Cover the bowl and refrigerate overnight, or for at least 4 hours, allowing the chia seeds to absorb the liquid and create a pudding-like consistency.

3. Before serving, give the chia pudding a good stir to break up any clumps. Top with fresh berries and chopped nuts for added flavor and texture.

Energizing Quinoa Breakfast Bowl

Ingredients:

- 1/2 cup cooked quinoa
- 1/4 cup unsweetened almond milk
- 1 tablespoon almond butter
- 1 tablespoon pure maple syrup
- 1/2 teaspoon cinnamon
- Sliced banana, for topping
- Chopped nuts, for topping

Instructions:

1. In a saucepan, warm the cooked quinoa with almond milk over medium heat until heated through.

2. Stir in the almond butter, maple syrup, and cinnamon, ensuring that everything is well combined.

3. Transfer the quinoa mixture to a bowl and top with sliced banana and chopped nuts. Enjoy this energizing breakfast bowl that is packed with protein and healthy fats.

Turmeric Ginger Smoothie Bowl

Ingredients:

- 1 frozen banana
- 1 cup frozen mango chunks
- 1 cup spinach
- 1/2 teaspoon turmeric powder
- 1/2-inch piece of fresh ginger, peeled
- 1 tablespoon chia seeds
- 1 cup unsweetened almond milk
- Toppings of your choice (e.g., sliced almonds, shredded coconut, berries)

Instructions:

1. In a blender, combine the frozen banana, frozen mango chunks, spinach, turmeric powder, fresh ginger, chia seeds, and almond milk. Blend until smooth and creamy.

2. Pour the smoothie into a bowl and add your desired toppings, such as sliced almonds, shredded coconut, or fresh berries. This vibrant and nutritious turmeric ginger smoothie bowl will leave you feeling refreshed and ready to tackle the day.

Gut-Nourishing Avocado Toast

Ingredients:

- 2 slices of whole-grain bread
- 1 ripe avocado
- Juice of half a lemon
- Salt and pepper to taste
- Red pepper flakes (optional)
- Fresh cilantro, for garnish

Instructions:

1. Toast the slices of bread to your desired level of
   crispiness.

2. In a bowl, mash the ripe avocado with the lemon
   juice, salt, and pepper until smooth and well
   combined.

3. Spread the avocado mixture evenly onto the toasted
   bread slices.

4. Sprinkle with red pepper flakes for an extra kick, if
   desired, and garnish with fresh cilantro. Indulge in
   this simple yet satisfying gut-nourishing avocado
   toast.

Berry and Kale Breakfast Smoothie

Ingredients:

- 1 cup kale leaves, stems removed
- 1/2 cup frozen mixed berries (e.g., strawberries, blueberries, raspberries)
- 1 ripe banana
- 1 tablespoon almond butter
- 1 cup unsweetened almond milk

- 1 tablespoon honey or agave syrup (optional, for added sweetness)

Instructions:

1. In a blender, combine the kale leaves, frozen mixed berries, ripe banana, almond butter, almond milk, and sweetener if desired. Blend until smooth and creamy.

2. Pour the smoothie into a glass and enjoy this antioxidant-rich and refreshing breakfast option that will help nourish your gut and provide a boost of vitamins and minerals.

Gut-Friendly Vegetable Omelet

Ingredients:

- 3 large eggs
- 1/4 cup diced bell peppers (any color)
- 1/4 cup diced zucchini
- 1/4 cup diced mushrooms
- 1/4 cup chopped spinach
- Salt and pepper to taste

- 1 tablespoon olive oil

Instructions:

1. In a bowl, whisk the eggs until well beaten. Season
    with salt and pepper.
2. Heat the olive oil in a non-stick skillet over medium
    heat.
3. Add the diced bell peppers, zucchini, mushrooms,
    and spinach to the skillet. Sauté for a few minutes
    until the vegetables are tender.
4. Pour the beaten eggs over the sautéed vegetables
    and cook until the omelet is set, about 3-4 minutes.
5. Gently fold the omelet in half and transfer it to a
    plate. Serve this gut-friendly vegetable omelet hot
    and savor the flavors of the fresh vegetables.

Buckwheat Pancakes with Blueberry Compote

Ingredients:

- 1 cup buckwheat flour
- 1 tablespoon coconut sugar

- 1 teaspoon baking powder
- 1/4 teaspoon salt
- 1 cup almond milk
- 1 large egg
- 1 tablespoon coconut oil, melted
- Fresh blueberries, for topping

Instructions:

1. In a bowl, whisk together the buckwheat flour, coconut sugar, baking powder, and salt.
2. In a separate bowl, whisk together the almond milk, egg, and melted coconut oil.
3. Pour the wet ingredients into the dry ingredients and stir until just combined. Do not overmix; a few lumps are okay.
4. Heat a non-stick skillet or griddle over medium heat and lightly grease it with coconut oil or cooking spray.
5. Pour 1/4 cup of the batter onto the skillet for each pancake. Cook until bubbles form on the surface, then flip and cook the other side until golden brown.

6. Repeat with the remaining batter. Serve the
    buckwheat pancakes topped with fresh blueberries
    and a drizzle of blueberry compote for a delightful
    and nutritious breakfast treat.

Spinach and Mushroom Frittata

Ingredients:

- 6 large eggs
- 1 cup fresh spinach leaves
- 1 cup sliced mushrooms
- 1/4 cup diced onion
- 1/4 cup shredded cheddar cheese
- Salt and pepper to taste
- 1 tablespoon olive oil

Instructions:

1. Preheat the oven to 350°F (175°C).
2. In a bowl, whisk the eggs and season with salt and
    pepper.
3. Heat the olive oil in an oven-safe skillet over
    medium heat.

4. Sauté the spinach, mushrooms, and onion in the skillet until the vegetables are tender.

5. Pour the whisked eggs over the sautéed vegetables in the skillet, ensuring they are evenly distributed.

6. Sprinkle the shredded cheddar cheese over the top.

7. Transfer the skillet to the preheated oven and bake for25-30 minutes or until the frittata is set in the center and the top is golden brown.

8. Remove the skillet from the oven and let it cool slightly before slicing and serving. This spinach and mushroom frittata is a fantastic option for a protein-packed breakfast that will keep you satisfied and nourished.

Gut-Soothing Acai Bowl

Ingredients:

- 2 frozen acai packets
- 1/2 cup frozen mixed berries
- 1 ripe banana
- 1/4 cup unsweetened almond milk

- Toppings of your choice (e.g., sliced banana, granola, coconut flakes)

Instructions:

1. In a blender, combine the frozen acai packets, frozen mixed berries, ripe banana, and almond milk. Blend until smooth and creamy.
2. Pour the acai mixture into a bowl and add your desired toppings, such as sliced banana, granola, or coconut flakes. This gut-soothing acai bowl is not only visually appealing but also loaded with antioxidants and fiber to support your digestive health.

Cinnamon Apple Quinoa Porridge

Ingredients:

- 1 cup cooked quinoa
- 1 cup unsweetened almond milk
- 1 apple, diced
- 1 tablespoon pure maple syrup
- 1/2 teaspoon cinnamon

- Chopped nuts, for topping

Instructions:

1. In a saucepan, combine the cooked quinoa, almond milk, diced apple, maple syrup, and cinnamon. Stir well.

2. Heat the mixture over medium heat, stirring occasionally, until the porridge is heated through and the apple is tender.

3. Remove from heat and let it cool slightly before serving.

4. Sprinkle with chopped nuts for added crunch and enjoy this cinnamon apple quinoa porridge that is both satisfying and nutritious.

Zucchini and Sweet Potato Breakfast Hash

Ingredients:

- 1 medium zucchini, diced
- 1 small sweet potato, peeled and diced
- 1/4 cup diced onion

- 2 cloves garlic, minced
- 1 tablespoon olive oil
- Salt and pepper to taste
- Fresh parsley, for garnish

Instructions:

1. Heat the olive oil in a skillet over medium heat.
2. Add the diced zucchini, sweet potato, onion, and minced garlic to the skillet. Sauté until the vegetables are tender and lightly browned.
3. Season with salt and pepper to taste.
4. Transfer the breakfast hash to a plate and garnish with fresh parsley. This zucchini and sweet potato breakfast hash is a fantastic way to incorporate vegetables into your morning routine while supporting your gut health.

Chapter 3: Lunch Recipes

In this chapter, we will explore a variety of delicious and nourishing lunch recipes that are specifically designed to promote gut health. Each recipe incorporates wholesome ingredients and flavors to support your well-being.

Gut-Healing Chicken and Vegetable Stir-Fry

Ingredients:

- 2 boneless, skinless chicken breasts, thinly sliced
- 2 tablespoons olive oil
- 1 red bell pepper, sliced
- 1 yellow bell pepper, sliced
- 1 cup broccoli florets
- 1 cup snap peas
- 2 cloves garlic, minced
- 1-inch piece of ginger, grated
- 2 tablespoons tamari or soy sauce
- 1 tablespoon honey or maple syrup
- 1 tablespoon apple cider vinegar

- 2 green onions, sliced
- Sesame seeds, for garnish

Instructions:

1. Heat 1 tablespoon of olive oil in a large skillet or wok over medium-high heat.
2. Add the chicken slices and cook until browned and cooked through. Remove the chicken from the skillet and set aside.
3. In the same skillet, add the remaining tablespoon of olive oil and sauté the bell peppers, broccoli, snap peas, garlic, and ginger for 4-5 minutes, or until the vegetables are crisp-tender.
4. In a small bowl, whisk together the tamari or soy sauce, honey or maple syrup, and apple cider vinegar.
5. Pour the sauce over the vegetables in the skillet and stir to coat evenly.
6. Add the cooked chicken back to the skillet and toss everything together for another 2-3 minutes, until heated through.

7. Remove from heat and garnish with sliced green onions and sesame seeds.

8. Serve the stir-fry hot and enjoy its gut-healing goodness.

Quinoa Salad with Roasted Vegetables

Ingredients:

- 1 cup quinoa, rinsed
- 2 cups vegetable broth or water
- 1 small butternut squash, peeled, seeded, and diced
- 1 red onion, sliced
- 1 red bell pepper, sliced
- 1 yellow bell pepper, sliced
- 1 zucchini, sliced
- 2 tablespoons olive oil
- 1 teaspoon cumin
- 1 teaspoon paprika
- Salt and pepper to taste
- Juice of 1 lemon
- Fresh parsley, chopped, for garnish

Instructions:

1. Preheat the oven to 400°F (200°C).

2. In a saucepan, combine the quinoa and vegetable broth or water. Bring to a boil, then reduce heat, cover, and simmer for 15-20 minutes until the quinoa is tender and the liquid is absorbed. Remove from heat and let it cool.

3. In a large mixing bowl, toss the diced butternut squash, red onion, red and yellow bell peppers, and zucchini with olive oil, cumin, paprika, salt, and pepper.

4. Spread the vegetables evenly on a baking sheet and roast in the preheated oven for 25-30 minutes, or until they are tender and slightly caramelized.

5. In a separate bowl, whisk together the lemon juice, olive oil, salt, and pepper to create the dressing.

6. In a large serving bowl, combine the cooked quinoa, roasted vegetables, and dressing. Mix well to ensure the flavors are evenly distributed.

7. Garnish with fresh parsley and serve the quinoa salad either warm or chilled.

Gut-Nourishing Greek Salad

Ingredients:

- 2 large cucumbers, diced
- 2 cups cherry tomatoes, halved
- 1 red onion, thinly sliced
- 1 green bell pepper, diced
- 1 cup Kalamata olives, pitted
- 1 cup feta cheese, crumbled
- ¼ cup extra-virgin olive oil
- 2 tablespoons red wine vinegar
- 1 teaspoon dried oregano
- Salt and pepper to taste
- Fresh parsley, chopped, for garnish

Instructions:

1. In a large bowl, combine the diced cucumbers, cherry tomatoes, red onion, green bell pepper, Kalamata olives, and crumbled feta cheese.

2. In a small bowl, whisk together the extra-virgin olive oil, red wine vinegar, dried oregano, salt, and pepper to make the dressing.

3. Pour the dressing over the salad ingredients and toss gently to combine.

4. Let the Greek salad sit at room temperature for 15-20 minutes to allow the flavors to meld together.

5. Garnish with fresh parsley and serve this gut-nourishing salad as a light and refreshing lunch option.

Gut-Friendly Lentil Soup

Ingredients:

- 1 cup dried green lentils, rinsed
- 1 tablespoon olive oil
- 1 onion, diced
- 2 carrots, diced
- 2 celery stalks, diced
- 3 cloves garlic, minced
- 1 teaspoon cumin
- 1 teaspoon paprika
- 4 cups vegetable broth
- 1 bay leaf
- Salt and pepper to taste
- Fresh cilantro, chopped, for garnish

Instructions:

1. Heat the olive oil in a large pot over medium heat.

2. Add the diced onion, carrots, and celery to the pot and sauté for 5-7 minutes until they begin to soften.

3. Stir in the minced garlic, cumin, and paprika, and cook for an additional minute until fragrant.

4. Add the rinsed lentils, vegetable broth, bay leaf, salt, and pepper to the pot. Stir well to combine.

5. Bring the soup to a boil, then reduce the heat to low, cover, and simmer for 30-35 minutes, or until the lentils are tender.

6. Remove the bay leaf from the soup and adjust the seasoning if needed.

7. Ladle the gut-friendly lentil soup into bowls, garnish with fresh cilantro, and serve hot. Enjoy its comforting flavors and nourishing properties.

Mediterranean Chickpea Salad

Ingredients:

- 2 cans chickpeas, drained and rinsed
- 1 cucumber, diced
- 1 red bell pepper, diced

- 1 cup cherry tomatoes, halved
- ½ red onion, thinly sliced
- ½ cup Kalamata olives, pitted and halved
- ½ cup crumbled feta cheese
- ¼ cup fresh parsley, chopped
- ¼ cup fresh mint, chopped
- 2 tablespoons extra-virgin olive oil
- 1 tablespoon lemon juice
- 1 teaspoon dried oregano
- Salt and pepper to taste

Instructions:

1. In a large bowl, combine the chickpeas, diced cucumber, red bell pepper, cherry tomatoes, red onion, Kalamata olives, crumbled feta cheese, fresh parsley, and fresh mint.

2. In a small bowl, whisk together the extra-virgin olive oil, lemon juice, dried oregano, salt, and pepper to create the dressing.

3. Drizzle the dressing over the salad ingredients and toss gently to coat everything evenly.

4. Allow the Mediterranean chickpea saladto sit for about 10-15 minutes to allow the flavors to meld together.

5. Serve the salad as a satisfying and protein-packed lunch option. Its vibrant colors and Mediterranean flavors will surely delight your taste buds.

Gut-Soothing Salmon and Asparagus Parcels

Ingredients:

- 2 salmon fillets
- 1 bunch asparagus, trimmed
- 1 lemon, thinly sliced
- 2 cloves garlic, minced
- 2 tablespoons fresh dill, chopped
- 2 tablespoons extra-virgin olive oil
- Salt and pepper to taste

Instructions:

1. Preheat the oven to 400°F (200°C).

2. Cut two large pieces of aluminum foil, enough to wrap each salmon fillet and asparagus.

3. Place a salmon fillet in the center of each foil piece.

4. Arrange a handful of trimmed asparagus spears next to each salmon fillet.

5. Sprinkle minced garlic and fresh dill over the salmon and asparagus.

6. Drizzle extra-virgin olive oil over the ingredients and season with salt and pepper to taste.

7. Place a few lemon slices on top of each salmon fillet.

8. Fold the sides of the foil over the salmon and asparagus, sealing the edges tightly to create a parcel.

9. Transfer the foil parcels to a baking sheet and bake in the preheated oven for 12-15 minutes, or until the salmon is cooked through and the asparagus is tender.

10. Carefully open the foil parcels, being cautious of the steam, and transfer the salmon and asparagus to serving plates.

11. Serve the gut-soothing salmon and asparagus parcels with a side of brown rice or quinoa for a complete and nourishing lunch.

Gut-Healthy Turkey and Vegetable Wrap

Ingredients:

- 4 large whole wheat tortilla wraps
- 8 slices of roasted turkey breast
- 1 cup baby spinach leaves
- 1 large tomato, thinly sliced
- 1 cucumber, thinly sliced
- 4 tablespoons hummus
- 2 tablespoons Dijon mustard
- Salt and pepper to taste

Instructions:

1. Lay out the whole wheat tortilla wraps on a clean surface.
2. Spread 1 tablespoon of hummus on each tortilla, leaving a border around the edges.
3. Drizzle ½ tablespoon of Dijon mustard over the hummus on each wrap.
4. Layer 2 slices of roasted turkey breast, a handful of baby spinach leaves, tomato slices, and cucumber slices on each wrap.

5. Season with salt and pepper to taste.

6. Fold the sides of the tortilla wraps inward and roll them tightly to form a secure wrap.

7. Slice the wraps in half diagonally and serve them as a gut-healthy and satisfying lunch option. Enjoy their fresh and flavorful combination.

Spinach and Feta Stuffed Bell Peppers

Ingredients:

- 4 bell peppers (any color), tops removed and seeds removed
- 1 tablespoon olive oil
- 1 onion, diced
- 2 cloves garlic, minced
- 4 cups baby spinach
- 1 cup crumbled feta cheese
- ½ cup cooked quinoa
- 1 teaspoon dried oregano
- Salt and pepper to taste

Instructions:

1. Preheat the oven to 375°F (190°C).

2. In a large pot of boiling water, blanch the bell peppers for 3-4 minutes until slightly softened. Remove them from the water and set aside.

3. Heat the olive oil in a skillet over medium heat.

4. Add the diced onion and minced garlic to the skillet and sauté for 2-3 minutes until softened and fragrant.

5. Add the baby spinach to the skillet and cook until wilted, stirring occasionally.

6. Remove the skillet from heat and stir in the crumbled feta cheese, cooked quinoa, dried oregano, salt, and pepper. Mix well to combine.

7. Stuff each bell pepper with the spinach and feta mixture, packing it tightly.

8. Place the stuffed bell peppers in a baking dish and bake in the preheated oven for 25-30 minutes, or until the peppers are tender and the filling is heated through.

9. Remove the dish from the oven and let the stuffed bell peppers cool slightly before serving.

10. These spinach and feta stuffed bell peppers make
for a wholesome and flavorful lunch option, packed
with nutrients to support your gut health.

Gut-Healing Sweet Potato and Black Bean Burrito Bowl

Ingredients:

- 2 medium sweet potatoes, peeled and diced
- 1 tablespoon olive oil
- 1 teaspoon chili powder
- ½ teaspoon cumin
- Salt and pepper to taste
- 1 can black beans, drained and rinsed
- 1 cup cooked brown rice
- 1 cup cherry tomatoes, halved
- ½ red onion, diced
- 1 jalapeno pepper, seeds removed and diced (optional)
- ¼ cup fresh cilantro, chopped
- Juice of 1 lime
- Greek yogurt or sour cream (optional), for serving

Instructions:

1. Preheat the oven to 400°F (200°C).
2. In a large bowl, toss the diced sweet potatoes with olive oil, chili powder, cumin, salt, and pepper until evenly coated.
3. Spread the seasoned sweet potatoes on a baking sheet and roast in the preheated oven for 25-30 minutes, or until they are tender and slightly caramelized.
4. In a separate bowl, combine the black beans, cooked brown rice, cherry tomatoes, diced red onion, diced jalapeno pepper (if using), chopped cilantro, and lime juice. Mix well.
5. Once the sweet potatoes are roasted, add them to the black bean and rice mixture and toss gently to combine.
6. Divide the burrito bowl mixture into serving bowls.
7. Serve the gut-healing sweet potato and black bean burrito bowl with a dollop of Greek yogurt or sour cream, if desired. Its vibrant colors and robust flavors make it a satisfying lunch option.

Butternut Squash and Quinoa Stuffed Portobello Mushrooms

Ingredients:

- 4 large Portobello mushrooms, stems removed
- 1 butternut squash, peeled, seeded, and diced
- 2 tablespoons olive oil
- 1 onion, diced
- 2 cloves garlic, minced
- 1 cup cooked quinoa
- ½ cup dried cranberries
- ½ cup crumbled goat cheese
- ¼ cup fresh sage leaves, chopped
- Salt and pepper to taste

Instructions:

1. Preheat the oven to 375°F (190°C).
2. Place the Portobello mushrooms on a baking sheet, gill-side up.
3. In a large bowl, toss the diced butternut squash with olive oil, salt, and pepper until coated.

4. Spread the butternut squash evenly on a separate baking sheet and roast in the preheated oven for 20-25 minutes, or until tender and golden.

5. In a skillet, heat the olive oil over medium heat.

6. Add the diced onion and minced garlic to the skillet and sauté until softened and fragrant.

7. Stir in the cooked quinoa, dried cranberries, crumbledgoat cheese, chopped fresh sage leaves, roasted butternut squash, salt, and pepper. Mix well to combine.

8. Spoon the quinoa and butternut squash mixture into the gill-side of each Portobello mushroom, filling them generously.

9. Return the mushrooms to the oven and bake for an additional 15-20 minutes, or until the mushrooms are tender and the filling is heated through.

10. Remove the stuffed Portobello mushrooms from the oven and let them cool slightly before serving.

11. These butternut squash and quinoa stuffed Portobello mushrooms make for a flavorful and satisfying lunch option. The combination of textures and flavors will surely impress your taste buds.

Gut-Nourishing Cauliflower Rice Sushi Rolls

Ingredients:

- 2 cups cauliflower rice
- 4 nori seaweed sheets
- 8 cooked shrimp, peeled and deveined
- 1 avocado, sliced
- 1 cucumber, julienned
- 2 tablespoons low-sodium soy sauce
- 1 tablespoon rice vinegar
- 1 tablespoon sesame oil
- Pickled ginger and wasabi, for serving (optional)

Instructions:

1. Place the cauliflower rice in a microwave-safe bowl and microwave for 3-4 minutes until cooked through. Let it cool slightly.
2. Lay a nori seaweed sheet on a clean surface, shiny side down.
3. Spread an even layer of cauliflower rice on the bottom two-thirds of the nori sheet, leaving a small border at the top.

4. Place two cooked shrimp, avocado slices, and julienned cucumber on top of the cauliflower rice.

5. Drizzle low-sodium soy sauce, rice vinegar, and sesame oil over the filling.

6. Using a sushi mat or your hands, tightly roll the nori sheet from the bottom, applying gentle pressure to form a compact sushi roll.

7. Repeat the process with the remaining nori sheets and filling ingredients.

8. Slice each sushi roll into bite-sized pieces using a sharp knife.

9. Serve the gut-nourishing cauliflower rice sushi rolls with pickled ginger and wasabi, if desired. Their light and fresh flavors make them a perfect lunchtime treat.

Chapter 4: Dinner Recipes

Gut-Friendly Grilled Salmon with Lemon and Dill

Ingredients:

- 4 salmon fillets
- 2 lemons, sliced
- Fresh dill, chopped
- Salt and pepper to taste
- Olive oil

Instructions:

1. Preheat the grill to medium-high heat.
2. Season the salmon fillets with salt and pepper.
3. Drizzle olive oil on both sides of the salmon.
4. Place the salmon fillets on the grill, skin side down.
5. Grill for about 4-5 minutes on each side or until the salmon is cooked through.
6. Squeeze fresh lemon juice over the grilled salmon.
7. Sprinkle chopped dill on top.

8. Serve the grilled salmon with lemon slices and garnish with additional dill.

Gut-Soothing Roasted Chicken with Herbs

Ingredients:

- 4 chicken breasts
- 2 tablespoons olive oil
- 2 cloves garlic, minced
- 1 teaspoon dried thyme
- 1 teaspoon dried rosemary
- Salt and pepper to taste

Instructions:

1. Preheat the oven to 400°F (200°C).
2. Rub the chicken breasts with olive oil, garlic, thyme, rosemary, salt, and pepper.
3. Place the chicken breasts in a baking dish.
4. Roast in the preheated oven for 20-25 minutes or until the chicken is cooked through.
5. Remove from the oven and let it rest for a few minutes before serving.

6. Slice the roasted chicken and serve with your choice of side dishes.

Gut-Nourishing Quinoa-Stuffed Bell Peppers

Ingredients:

- 4 bell peppers (any color)
- 1 cup cooked quinoa
- 1 cup black beans, rinsed and drained
- 1 cup corn kernels
- 1 small onion, finely chopped
- 2 cloves garlic, minced
- 1 teaspoon ground cumin
- 1 teaspoon paprika
- Salt and pepper to taste
- Fresh cilantro, chopped (for garnish)

Instructions:

1. Preheat the oven to 375°F (190°C).
2. Cut off the tops of the bell peppers and remove the seeds and membranes.

3. In a large bowl, combine cooked quinoa, black beans, corn, onion, garlic, cumin, paprika, salt, and pepper. Mix well.

4. Stuff the bell peppers with the quinoa mixture and place them in a baking dish.

5. Cover the dish with foil and bake for 30-35 minutes or until the bell peppers are tender.

6. Remove from the oven and garnish with fresh cilantro before serving.

Gut-Healing Shrimp and Vegetable Stir-Fry

Ingredients:

- 1 pound shrimp, peeled and deveined
- 2 tablespoons olive oil
- 2 cloves garlic, minced
- 1 teaspoon grated ginger
- 1 bell pepper, thinly sliced
- 1 zucchini, sliced
- 1 carrot, sliced
- 1 cup broccoli florets

- 2 tablespoons soy sauce (or tamari for a gluten-free option)
- 1 tablespoon honey (or maple syrup for a vegan option)
- Salt and pepper to taste
- Sesame seeds (for garnish)

Instructions:

1. Heat olive oil in a large skillet or wok over medium heat.
2. Add garlic and ginger and cook for about 1 minute until fragrant.
3. Add the shrimp to the skillet and cook until they turn pink and opaque.
4. Remove the shrimp from the skillet and set aside.
5. In the same skillet, add the bell pepper, zucchini, carrot, and broccoli. Stir-fry for about 3-4 minutes until the vegetables are tender-crisp.
6. In a small bowl, whisk together soy sauce and honey. Pour the sauce into the skillet with the vegetables.

7. Return the shrimp to the skillet and toss everything together to coat in the sauce.

8. Season with salt and pepper to taste.

9. Garnish with sesame seeds before serving.

Gut-Friendly Lentil Curry

Ingredients:

- 1 cup dried lentils
- 2 tablespoons olive oil
- 1 onion, chopped
- 2 cloves garlic, minced
- 1 tablespoon curry powder
- 1 teaspoon ground cumin
- 1 teaspoon ground turmeric
- 1 can (14 ounces) diced tomatoes
- 1 can (14 ounces) coconut milk
- Salt and pepper to taste
- Fresh cilantro, chopped (for garnish)

Instructions:

1. Rinse the lentils under cold water and drain.

2. In a large pot, heat olive oil over medium heat.

3. Add the onion and garlic and sauté until softened.

4. Stir in curry powder, cumin, and turmeric and cook for 1 minute until fragrant.

5. Add the lentils, diced tomatoes (with their juices), and coconut milk to the pot. Stir well.

6. Bring the mixture to a boil, then reduce the heat and simmer for about 25-30 minutes or until the lentils are tender.

7. Season with salt and pepper to taste.

8. Garnish with fresh cilantro before serving.

9. Serve the lentil curry with rice or naan bread.

Gut-Soothing Sweet Potato and Chickpea Curry

Ingredients:

- 2 tablespoons olive oil
- 1 onion, chopped
- 2 cloves garlic, minced
- 1 tablespoon grated ginger
- 1 teaspoon ground cumin
- 1 teaspoon ground coriander
- 1 teaspoon turmeric

- 1 teaspoon paprika
- 1 sweet potato, peeled and cubed
- 1 can (14 ounces) chickpeas, rinsed and drained
- 1 can (14 ounces) diced tomatoes
- 1 can (14 ounces) coconut milk
- Salt and pepper to taste
- Fresh cilantro, chopped (for garnish)

Instructions:

1. Heat olive oil in a large pot over medium heat.
2. Add the onion, garlic, and ginger to the pot and sauté until the onion is translucent.
3. Stir in cumin, coriander, turmeric, and paprika. Cook for 1 minute until fragrant.
4. Add the sweet potato, chickpeas, diced tomatoes (with their juices), and coconut milk to the pot. Stir well.
5. Bring the mixture to a boil, then reduce the heat and simmer for about 20-25 minutes or until the sweet potato is tender.
6. Season with salt and pepper to taste.
7. Garnish with fresh cilantro before serving.

8. Serve the sweet potato and chickpea curry with rice or naan bread.

Gut-Healthy Turkey Meatballs with Zucchini Noodles

Ingredients:

- 1 pound ground turkey
- 1/2 cup almond flour
- 1/4 cup grated Parmesan cheese
- 1 egg
- 2 cloves garlic, minced
- 1 teaspoon dried oregano
- 1 teaspoon dried basil
- 1/2 teaspoon salt
- 1/4 teaspoon black pepper
- 2 tablespoons olive oil
- 4 medium zucchini,sliced into noodles (using a spiralizer or julienne peeler)
- 2 cups marinara sauce
- Fresh basil, chopped (for garnish)

Instructions:

1. In a large bowl, combine ground turkey, almond flour, Parmesan cheese, egg, garlic, oregano, basil, salt, and pepper. Mix well.

2. Shape the mixture into meatballs, about 1 inch in diameter.

3. Heat olive oil in a large skillet over medium heat.

4. Add the meatballs to the skillet and cook until browned on all sides and cooked through, about 10-12 minutes.

5. Remove the meatballs from the skillet and set aside.

6. In the same skillet, add the zucchini noodles and cook for about 2-3 minutes until slightly softened.

7. Pour the marinara sauce into the skillet with the zucchini noodles and stir well.

8. Return the meatballs to the skillet and simmer for another 2-3 minutes to heat through.

9. Garnish with fresh basil before serving.

Gut-Nourishing Baked Cod with Garlic and Herbs

Ingredients:

- 4 cod fillets

- 2 tablespoons olive oil

- 4 cloves garlic, minced

- 1 tablespoon fresh parsley, chopped

- 1 tablespoon fresh dill, chopped

- 1 tablespoon fresh lemon juice

- Salt and pepper to taste

- Lemon wedges (for serving)

Instructions:

1. Preheat the oven to 400°F (200°C).

2. Place the cod fillets in a baking dish.

3. In a small bowl, combine olive oil, minced garlic, parsley, dill, lemon juice, salt, and pepper. Mix well.

4. Drizzle the garlic and herb mixture over the cod fillets, making sure they are evenly coated.

5. Bake in the preheated oven for 12-15 minutes or until the cod is opaque and flakes easily with a fork.

6. Remove from the oven and let it rest for a few minutes before serving.

7. Serve the baked cod with lemon wedges.

Gut-Healing Stuffed Cabbage Rolls

Ingredients:

- 1 large head of cabbage
- 1 pound ground beef (or turkey)
- 1 cup cooked quinoa
- 1 small onion, finely chopped
- 2 cloves garlic, minced
- 1 can (14 ounces) diced tomatoes
- 1 can (14 ounces) tomato sauce
- 1 teaspoon dried oregano
- 1 teaspoon dried basil
- Salt and pepper to taste
- Fresh parsley, chopped (for garnish)

Instructions:

1. Preheat the oven to 350°F (175°C).
2. Remove the core from the cabbage and place the whole head in a large pot of boiling water.
3. Boil for about 5 minutes until the outer leaves become pliable. Carefully remove the leaves and set them aside to cool.

4. In a large bowl, combine ground beef, cooked quinoa, onion, garlic, oregano, basil, salt, and pepper. Mix well.

5. Take a cabbage leaf and place a small amount of the meat mixture in the center. Roll the leaf, tucking in the sides, to form a cabbage roll. Repeat with the remaining leaves and meat mixture.

6. In a baking dish, spread a thin layer of diced tomatoes and tomato sauce.

7. Place the cabbage rolls in the baking dish, seam side down.

8. Pour the remaining diced tomatoes and tomato sauce over the cabbage rolls.

9. Cover the baking dish with foil and bake for 45-50 minutes or until the cabbage rolls are cooked through.

10. Garnish with fresh parsley before serving.

Gut-Friendly Vegetarian Chili

Ingredients:

- 1 tablespoon olive oil
- 1 onion, chopped

- 2 cloves garlic, minced
- 1 bell pepper, diced
- 1 zucchini, diced
- 1 carrot, diced
- 1 can (14 ounces) diced tomatoes
- 1 can (14 ounces) kidney beans, rinsed and drained
- 1 can (14 ounces) black beans, rinsed and drained
- 1 cup vegetable broth
- 2 tablespoons chili powder
- 1 teaspoon cumin
- 1 teaspoon paprika
- Salt and pepper to taste
- Fresh cilantro, chopped (for garnish)

Instructions:

1. Heat olive oil in a large pot over medium heat.
2. Add the onion and garlic to the pot and sauté until the onion is translucent.
3. Add the bell pepper, zucchini, and carrot to the pot and cook for about 5 minutes until the vegetables start to soften.

4. Stir in diced tomatoes, kidney beans, black beans, vegetable broth, chili powder, cumin, paprika, salt, and pepper. Mix well.

5. Bring the chili to a boil, then reduce the heat and simmer for about 30-40 minutes to allow the flavors to meld together.

6. Season with additional salt and pepper if needed.

7. Garnish with fresh cilantro before serving.

8. Serve the vegetarian chili with your choice of toppings, such as avocado slices or shredded cheese.

Gut-Soothing Moroccan Vegetable Tagine

Ingredients:

- 2 tablespoons olive oil
- 1 onion, chopped
- 2 cloves garlic, minced
- 1 teaspoon grated ginger
- 1 teaspoon ground cumin
- 1 teaspoon ground coriander
- 1 teaspoon ground turmeric

- 1/2 teaspoon ground cinnamon
- 1 sweet potato, peeled and cubed
- 2 carrots, sliced
- 1 zucchini, sliced
- 1 red bell pepper, sliced
- 1 can (14 ounces) diced tomatoes
- 1 cup vegetable broth
- 1/2 cup dried apricots, chopped
- Salt and pepper to taste
- Fresh cilantro, chopped (for garnish)

Instructions:

1. Heat olive oil in a large pot or tagine over medium heat.
2. Add the onion, garlic, and ginger to the pot and sauté until the onion is translucent.
3. Stir in cumin, coriander, turmeric, and cinnamon. Cook for 1 minute until fragrant.
4. Add the sweet potato, carrots, zucchini, red bell pepper, diced tomatoes (with their juices), vegetable broth, dried apricots, salt, and pepper to the pot. Stir well.

5. Bring the mixture to a boil, then reduce the heat to low and cover the pot.

6. Simmer for about 30-40 minutes or until the vegetables are tender.

7. Season with additional salt and pepper if needed.

8. Garnish with fresh cilantro before serving.

9. Serve the Moroccan vegetable tagine with couscous or quinoa.

Chapter 5: Snacks and Appetizers

In this chapter, we will explore a variety of delicious and gut-healthy snacks and appetizers that will not only satisfy your taste buds but also contribute to your overall well-being. These recipes are packed with wholesome ingredients that promote gut health and provide a satisfying and nutritious snack option.

Gut-Healing Turmeric Hummus with Veggie Sticks

Ingredients:

- 1 can of chickpeas, drained and rinsed
- 3 tablespoons of tahini
- 2 tablespoons of extra-virgin olive oil
- 2 cloves of garlic, minced
- 1 teaspoon of ground turmeric
- Juice of 1 lemon
- Salt and pepper to taste
- Assorted vegetable sticks (carrots, celery, bell peppers) for serving

Instructions:

1. In a food processor, combine the chickpeas, tahini, olive oil, garlic, turmeric, lemon juice, salt, and pepper.
2. Process the mixture until smooth and creamy, scraping down the sides as needed.
3. Taste and adjust the seasoning if needed.
4. Transfer the hummus to a serving bowl and serve with an assortment of vegetable sticks.

Gut-Nourishing Greek Yogurt Parfait with Berries

Ingredients:

- 1 cup of Greek yogurt
- 1 tablespoon of honey
- 1/2 teaspoon of vanilla extract
- 1/4 cup of granola
- 1/2 cup of mixed berries (strawberries, blueberries, raspberries)

Instructions:

1. In a bowl, combine the Greek yogurt, honey, and
   vanilla extract.

2. Mix well until the honey is evenly distributed.

3. In a glass or serving dish, layer the Greek yogurt
   mixture, granola, and mixed berries.

4. Repeat the layers until all the ingredients are used,
   finishing with a layer of berries on top.

5. Serve immediately or refrigerate until ready to
   enjoy.

Gut-Friendly Guacamole with Baked Tortilla Chips

Ingredients:

- 2 ripe avocados, peeled and pitted
- Juice of 1 lime
- 1/4 cup of red onion, finely chopped
- 1/4 cup of fresh cilantro, chopped
- 1 small tomato, diced
- 1 jalapeño pepper, seeded and minced
- Salt and pepper to taste
- Baked tortilla chips for serving

Instructions:

1. In a bowl, mash the avocados with a fork until smooth.

2. Add the lime juice and mix well to prevent browning.

3. Stir in the red onion, cilantro, tomato, and jalapeño pepper.

4. Season with salt and pepper, adjusting the flavors to your preference.

5. Transfer the guacamole to a serving bowl and serve with baked tortilla chips.

Gut-Soothing Cucumber and Tzatziki Bites

Ingredients:

*   1 English cucumber
*   1 cup of Greek yogurt
*   1/4 cup of fresh dill, chopped
*   1 clove of garlic, minced
*   Juice of 1/2 lemon
*   Salt and pepper to taste

Instructions:

1. Slice the cucumber into thick rounds.

2. In a bowl, combine the Greek yogurt, dill, garlic, lemon juice, salt, and pepper.

3. Mix well until all the ingredients are incorporated.

4. Place a dollop of the tzatziki mixture on each cucumber round.

5. Garnish with an extra sprinkle of dill.

6. Serve immediately and enjoy the refreshing and gut-soothing bites.

Gut-Healthy Almond and Date Energy Balls

Ingredients:

- 1 cup of almonds
- 1 cup of dates, pitted
- 2 tablespoons of unsweetened cocoa powder
- 1 tablespoon of chia seeds
- 1/2 teaspoon of vanilla extract
- Pinch of salt
- Shredded coconut (optional) for coating

Instructions:

1. In a food processor, blend the almonds until they form a coarse meal.

2. Add the dates, cocoa powder, chia seeds, vanilla extract, and salt to the food processor.

3. Process the mixture until it comes together and forms a sticky dough.

4. Roll the dough into small balls, about 1 inch in diameter.

5. If desired, roll the energy balls in shredded coconut for an additional touch of flavor.

6. Place the energy balls in an airtight container and refrigerate for at least 30 minutes before serving.

Gut-Nourishing Roasted Beetroot and Goat Cheese Crostini

Ingredients:

- 2 medium-sized beetroots, peeled and sliced
- 2 tablespoons of olive oil
- Salt and pepper to taste
- Baguette, sliced and toasted

- Goat cheese

- Fresh thyme leaves for garnish

Instructions:

1. Preheat the oven to 400°F (200°C).

2. In a bowl, toss the beetroot slices with olive oil, salt, and pepper.

3. Spread the beetroot slices on a baking sheet and roast for 20-25 minutes or until tender.

4. Remove the beetroot from the oven and let it cool slightly.

5. Spread goat cheese on each toasted baguette slice.

6. Top with a roasted beetroot slice and garnish with fresh thyme leaves.

7. Serve the crostini as a colorful and nourishing appetizer.

Gut-Healing Kale Chips

Ingredients:

- 1 bunch of kale, washed and dried

- 1 tablespoon of olive oil

- Salt and pepper to taste

Instructions:

1. Preheat the oven to 300°F (150°C).
2. Tear the kale leaves into bite-sized pieces, discarding the tough stems.
3. In a large bowl, toss the kale leaves with olive oil, salt, and pepper.
4. Spread the kale leaves in a single layer on a baking sheet.
5. Bake for 10-15 minutes or until the kale leaves are crispy but not burnt.
6. Remove from the oven and let them cool before serving.

Gut-Friendly Zucchini Fritters

Ingredients:

- 2 medium zucchinis, grated
- 1/2 teaspoon of salt
- 1/4 cup of chickpea flour
- 2 green onions, finely chopped
- 1/4 cup of fresh parsley, chopped

- 1 clove of garlic, minced
- 1/4 teaspoon of ground cumin
- 1/4 teaspoon of paprika
- 2 tablespoons of olive oil

Instructions:

1. Place the grated zucchinis in a colander and sprinkle with salt.
2. Let them sit for 10 minutes to release excess moisture.
3. Squeeze out any remaining moisture from the zucchini using a clean kitchen towel.
4. In a bowl, combine the zucchini, chickpea flour, green onions, parsley, garlic, cumin, and paprika.
5. Mix well until all the ingredients are evenly distributed.
6. Heat olive oil in a skillet over medium heat.
7. Spoon the zucchini mixture onto the skillet, forming small fritters.
8. Cook for 3-4 minutes per side or until golden brown.

Gut-Soothing Roasted Chickpeas with Spices

Ingredients:

- 1 can of chickpeas, drained and rinsed
- 1 tablespoon of olive oil
- 1 teaspoon of ground cumin
- 1/2 teaspoon of smoked paprika
- 1/2 teaspoon of garlic powder
- Salt and pepper to taste

Instructions:

1. Preheat the oven to 400°F (200°C).
2. Pat the chickpeas dry with a clean kitchen towel or paper towels.
3. In a bowl, toss the chickpeas with olive oil, cumin, smoked paprika, garlic powder, salt, and pepper.
4. Spread the chickpeas in a single layer on a baking sheet.
5. Roast in the preheated oven for 20-25 minutes or until crispy, shaking the pan occasionally to ensure even cooking.

6. Remove from the oven and let them cool slightly
    before serving.

Gut-Healthy Smoked Salmon Cucumber Roll-Ups

Ingredients:

- 1 English cucumber
- 4 ounces of smoked salmon
- 1/4 cup of cream cheese
- Fresh dill for garnish

Instructions:

1. Slice the cucumber lengthwise into thin strips using
    a vegetable peeler or a mandoline slicer.
2. Lay the cucumber slices flat on a clean surface.
3. Spread a thin layer of cream cheese on each
    cucumber slice.
4. Place a slice of smoked salmon on top of the cream
    cheese.
5. Roll up the cucumber slice tightly, securing it with a
    toothpick if needed.

6. Garnish with fresh dill.

7. Repeat the process with the remaining cucumber slices, smoked salmon, and cream cheese.

8. Serve the roll-ups as an elegant and gut-healthy appetizer.

Gut-Nourishing Stuffed Mushrooms with Spinach and Feta

Ingredients:

- 12 large mushrooms, stems removed
- 1 tablespoon of olive oil
- 2 cloves of garlic, minced
- 2 cups of fresh spinach, chopped
- 1/4 cup of crumbled feta cheese
- Salt and pepper to taste

Instructions:

1. Preheat the oven to 375°F (190°C).

2. Place the mushroom caps on a baking sheet, gill side up.

3. In a skillet, heat olive oil over medium heat.

4. Add the garlic and sauté for 1 minute until fragrant.

5. Add the chopped spinach and cook until wilted.

6. Remove the skillet from heat and let the mixture cool slightly.

7. Once cooled, stir in the feta cheese and season with salt and pepper.

8. Spoon the spinach and feta mixture into each mushroom cap, pressing gently.

9. Bake in the preheated oven for 15-20 minutes or until the mushrooms are tender.

10. Remove from the oven and let them cool for a few minutes before serving.

Chapter 6: Desserts

Gut-Healing Mixed Berry Parfait with Coconut Yogurt

Ingredients:

- 1 cup mixed berries (strawberries, blueberries, raspberries)
- 1 cup coconut yogurt
- 1 tablespoon honey or maple syrup
- 1/4 cup granola
- Fresh mint leaves for garnish (optional)

Instructions:

1. Wash and chop the berries into bite-sized pieces.
2. In a glass or parfait dish, layer a spoonful of coconut yogurt at the bottom.
3. Add a layer of mixed berries on top of the yogurt.
4. Drizzle a teaspoon of honey or maple syrup over the berries.
5. Repeat the layers until the glass or dish is filled, ending with a layer of berries on top.

6. Sprinkle granola over the final layer of berries.

7. Garnish with fresh mint leaves, if desired.

8. Serve immediately and enjoy the gut-healing goodness of this delicious parfait.

Gut-Nourishing Dark Chocolate Avocado Mousse

Ingredients:

- 2 ripe avocados
- 1/4 cup unsweetened cocoa powder
- 1/4 cup maple syrup or honey
- 1/4 cup almond milk (or any non-dairy milk)
- 1 teaspoon vanilla extract
- Fresh berries for garnish (optional)

Instructions:

1. Cut the avocados in half, remove the pits, and scoop out the flesh.

2. In a blender or food processor, combine the avocado flesh, cocoa powder, maple syrup or honey, almond milk, and vanilla extract.

3. Blend until smooth and creamy, scraping down the sides as needed.

4. Transfer the mixture to serving bowls or glasses.

5. Refrigerate for at least 1 hour to allow the mousse to set.

6. Garnish with fresh berries, if desired, before serving.

7. Indulge in this guilt-free, gut-nourishing dark chocolate avocado mousse.

Gut-Friendly Banana and Walnut Bread

Ingredients:

- 2 ripe bananas, mashed
- 1/2 cup coconut flour
- 1/2 cup almond flour
- 1/4 cup honey or maple syrup
- 1/4 cup coconut oil, melted
- 3 eggs
- 1 teaspoon baking powder
- 1/2 teaspoon cinnamon

- 1/4 teaspoon salt
- 1/2 cup chopped walnuts

Instructions:

1. Preheat the oven to 350°F (175°C) and grease a loaf pan.
2. In a large bowl, combine the mashed bananas, coconut flour, almond flour, honey or maple syrup, coconut oil, eggs, baking powder, cinnamon, and salt.
3. Mix well until all ingredients are fully incorporated.
4. Fold in the chopped walnuts.
5. Pour the batter into the greased loaf pan and spread it evenly.
6. Bake for 40-45 minutes or until a toothpick inserted into the center comes out clean.
7. Allow the banana and walnut bread to cool in the pan for 10 minutes, then transfer it to a wire rack to cool completely.
8. Slice and enjoy this gut-friendly and delicious bread as a dessert or snack.

Gut-Soothing Chia Seed Pudding with Mango

Ingredients:

- 1/4 cup chia seeds
- 1 cup coconut milk
- 1 tablespoon honey or maple syrup
- 1/2 teaspoon vanilla extract
- 1 ripe mango, diced
- Fresh mint leaves for garnish (optional)

Instructions:

1. In a bowl, combine the chia seeds, coconut milk, honey or maple syrup, and vanilla extract.
2. Stir well to ensure the chia seeds are evenly distributed.
3. Let the mixture sit for 5 minutes, then stir again to prevent clumping.
4. Cover the bowl and refrigerate for at least 2 hours or overnight, allowing the chia seeds to absorb the liquid and thicken.
5. Once the pudding has set, give it a good stir to break up any lumps.

6. Spoon the chia seed pudding into serving glasses or bowls.

7. Top with diced mango and garnish with fresh mint leaves, if desired.

8. Savor the gut-soothing goodness of this refreshing chia seed pudding with mango.

Gut-Healthy Blueberry Oat Bars

Ingredients:

- 2 cups rolled oats
- 1 cup almond flour
- 1/4 cup honey or maple syrup
- 1/4 cup coconut oil, melted
- 1/2 teaspoon vanilla extract
- 1/2 teaspoon cinnamon
- 1/4 teaspoon salt
- 1 cup fresh or frozen blueberries

Instructions:

1. Preheat the oven to 350°F (175°C) and grease a baking dish.

2. In a large bowl, combine the rolled oats, almond flour, honey or maple syrup, melted coconut oil, vanilla extract, cinnamon, and salt.

3. Mix until the ingredients are well combined and form a crumbly texture.

4. Set aside 1/2 cup of the mixture for the topping.

5. Press the remaining mixture into the greased baking dish, forming an even layer.

6. Spread the blueberries over the oat mixture in the baking dish.

7. Sprinkle the reserved oat mixture on top of the blueberries.

8. Bake for 30-35 minutes or until the edges are golden brown and the blueberries are bubbling.

9. Remove from the oven and let the bars cool completely before cutting into squares.

10. Enjoy these gut-healthy blueberry oat bars as a nutritious dessert or snack.

Gut-Nourishing Coconut Milk Rice Pudding

Ingredients:

- 1 cup white rice
- 2 cups coconut milk
- 1/4 cup honey or maple syrup
- 1/2 teaspoon vanilla extract
- 1/4 teaspoon ground cardamom
- 1/4 teaspoon salt
- 1/4 cup raisins or dried cranberries (optional)
- Shredded coconut for garnish (optional)

Instructions:

1. Rinse the rice under cold water until the water runs clear.
2. In a saucepan, combine the rinsed rice, coconut milk, honey or maple syrup, vanilla extract, ground cardamom, and salt.
3. Bring the mixture to a boil over medium heat.
4. Reduce the heat to low and simmer, covered, for 15-20 minutes or until the rice is tender and the liquid is absorbed, stirring occasionally.

5. If using, stir in the raisins or dried cranberries during the last few minutes of cooking.

6. Remove the rice pudding from the heat and let it sit, covered, for 5 minutes.

7. Fluff the rice pudding with a fork and transfer it to serving bowls.

8. Garnish with shredded coconut, if desired.

9. Allow the pudding to cool slightly before serving or refrigerate for a chilled dessert.

10. Indulge in this creamy and gut-nourishing coconut milk rice pudding.

Gut-Healing Baked Apples with Cinnamon and Almonds

Ingredients:

- 4 apples (Honeycrisp or Granny Smith work well)
- 1/4 cup chopped almonds
- 2 tablespoons honey or maple syrup
- 1 tablespoon coconut oil, melted
- 1 teaspoon ground cinnamon
- 1/4 teaspoon nutmeg

- 1/4 teaspoon salt
- Greek yogurt or coconut yogurt for serving (optional)

Instructions:

1. Preheat the oven to 375°F (190°C) and line a baking dish with parchment paper.
2. Core the apples using an apple corer or a knife, leaving the bottoms intact.
3. In a small bowl, combine the chopped almonds, honey or maple syrup, melted coconut oil, ground cinnamon, nutmeg, and salt.
4. Stuff each apple with the almond mixture, dividing it evenly among the apples.
5. Place the stuffed apples in the lined baking dish and cover with foil.
6. Bake for 25 minutes, then remove the foil and bake for an additional 10-15 minutes or until the apples are tender.
7. Remove from the oven and let the baked apples cool slightly.

8. Serve the baked apples warm, either on their own or with a dollop of Greek yogurt or coconut yogurt, if desired.

9. Enjoy the gut-healing benefits of these delicious baked apples with cinnamon and almonds.

Gut-Friendly Raspberry Coconut Ice Cream

Ingredients:

- 2 cups frozen raspberries
- 1 can (13.5 oz) full-fat coconut milk
- 1/4 cup honey or maple syrup
- 1 teaspoon vanilla extract
- Fresh raspberries for garnish (optional)

Instructions:

1. In a blender or food processor, combine the frozen raspberries, coconut milk, honey or maple syrup, and vanilla extract.

2. Blend until smooth and creamy, scraping down the sides as needed.

3. Transfer the mixture to an ice cream maker and churn according to the manufacturer's instructions.

4. Once the ice cream reaches a soft-serve consistency, transfer it to a lidded container and freeze for at least 2 hours to firm up.

5. Before serving, let the ice cream sit at room temperature for a few minutes to soften slightly.

6. Scoop the raspberry coconut ice cream into bowls or cones.

7. Garnish with fresh raspberries, if desired.

8. Enjoy this gut-friendly and refreshing raspberry coconut ice cream as a guilt-free dessert.

Gut-Soothing Pumpkin Spice Energy Bites

Ingredients:

- 1 cup rolled oats
- 1/2 cup pumpkin puree
- 1/4 cup almond butter
- 1/4 cup honey or maple syrup
- 1/4 cup ground flaxseed

- 1/4 cup chopped walnuts
- 1/4 cup dried cranberries or raisins
- 1 teaspoon pumpkin pie spice
- 1/2 teaspoon vanilla extract
- Shredded coconut for rolling (optional)

Instructions:

1. In a large bowl, combine the rolled oats, pumpkin puree, almond butter, honey or maple syrup, ground flaxseed, chopped walnuts, dried cranberries or raisins, pumpkin pie spice, and vanilla extract.
2. Stir until all ingredients are well combined and form a sticky mixture.
3. Place the bowl in the refrigerator for 15-30 minutes to allow the mixture to firm up slightly.
4. Once chilled, remove the bowl from the refrigerator.
5. Scoop tablespoon-sized portions of the mixture and roll them into balls using your hands.
6. If desired, roll the energy bites in shredded coconut for added flavor and texture.

7. Place the energy bites on a baking sheet lined with parchment paper.

8. Refrigerate for at least 1 hour to allow the energy bites to set.

9. Store in an airtight container in the refrigerator for up to one week.

10. Enjoy these gut-soothing pumpkin spice energy bites as a healthy snack or dessert.

Gut-Healthy Chocolate Chip Zucchini Bread

Ingredients:

- 2 cups shredded zucchini
- 1 3/4 cups whole wheat flour
- 1/2 cup coconut sugar or brown sugar
- 1/2 cup coconut oil, melted
- 1/4 cup almond milk (or any non-dairy milk)
- 2 eggs
- 1 teaspoon baking powder
- 1/2 teaspoon baking soda
- 1/2 teaspoon cinnamon

- 1/4 teaspoon salt
- 1/2 cup dark chocolate chips

Instructions:

1. Preheat the oven to 350°F (175°C) and grease a loaf pan.
2. Using a clean kitchen towel or paper towels, squeeze out any excess moisture from the shredded zucchini.
3. In a large bowl, combine the shredded zucchini, whole wheat flour, coconut sugar or brown sugar, melted coconut oil, almond milk, eggs, baking powder, baking soda, cinnamon, and salt.
4. Stir well until all ingredients are fully incorporated.
5. Fold in the dark chocolate chips.
6. Pour the batter into the greased loaf pan and spread it evenly.
7. Bake for 50-60 minutes or until a toothpick inserted into the center comes out clean.
8. Allow the zucchini bread to cool in the pan for 10 minutes, then transfer it to a wire rack to cool completely.

9. Slice and enjoy this gut-healthy chocolate chip zucchini bread as a delightful dessert or snack.

Gut-Nourishing Strawberry Chia Jam Thumbprint Cookies

Ingredients:

- 1 1/2 cups almond flour
- 1/4 cup coconut flour
- 1/4 cup coconut oil, melted
- 3 tablespoons honey or maple syrup
- 1 teaspoon vanilla extract
- 1/4 teaspoon salt
- 1/4 cup strawberry chia jam (store-bought or homemade)

Instructions:

1. Preheat the oven to 350°F (175°C) and line a baking sheet with parchment paper.
2. In a mixing bowl, combine the almond flour, coconut flour, melted coconut oil, honey or maple syrup, vanilla extract, and salt.

3. Stir until a dough forms.

4. Roll the dough into tablespoon-sized balls and place
    them on the prepared baking sheet.

5. Press your thumb into the center of each cookie to
    create an indentation.

6. Spoon a small amount of strawberry chia jam into
    each indentation.

7. Bake for 12-15 minutes or until the cookies are
    golden around the edges.

8. Remove from the oven and let the cookies cool on
    the baking sheet for a few minutes, then transfer
    them to a wire rack to cool completely.

9. Enjoy these gut-nourishing strawberry chia jam
    thumbprint cookies as a delightful treat.

Chapter 7: Smoothies

Smoothies are a fantastic way to incorporate a wide range of nutrients into your diet while enjoying a refreshing and delicious beverage. In this chapter, we will explore smoothie recipes specifically designed to support gut health.

Gut-Healing Green Detox Smoothie

Ingredients:

- 1 cup spinach
- 1 cup kale
- 1/2 cucumber, peeled and chopped
- 1 green apple, cored and chopped
- 1/2 lemon, juiced
- 1/2 inch ginger root, peeled
- 1 cup coconut water
- Ice cubes (optional)

Instructions:

1. Place all the ingredients in a blender.

2. Blend on high speed until smooth and creamy.

3. If desired, add ice cubes and blend again until well incorporated.

4. Pour into a glass and enjoy the refreshing taste of this gut-healing green detox smoothie.

Gut-Nourishing Berry Blast Smoothie

Ingredients:

- 1 cup mixed berries (strawberries, blueberries, raspberries)
- 1/2 cup Greek yogurt
- 1/2 cup almond milk
- 1 tablespoon chia seeds
- 1 tablespoon honey or maple syrup (optional)
- Ice cubes (optional)

Instructions:

1. Combine all the ingredients in a blender.

2. Blend until the mixture is smooth and creamy.

3. If desired, add ice cubes and blend again for a frostier texture.

4. Pour into a glass and savor the delightful flavors of this gut-nourishing berry blast smoothie.

Gut-Friendly Mango and Spinach Smoothie

Ingredients:

- 1 cup fresh or frozen mango chunks
- 1 cup spinach
- 1/2 banana
- 1/2 cup coconut water
- 1/2 cup almond milk
- 1 tablespoon flaxseeds
- Ice cubes (optional)

Instructions:

1. Place all the ingredients in a blender.

2. Blend until the mixture is creamy and well combined.

3. If desired, add ice cubes and blend again for a cooler consistency.

4. Pour into a glass and relish the tropical flavors of this gut-friendly mango and spinach smoothie.

Gut-Soothing Papaya and Pineapple Smoothie

Ingredients:

- 1 cup ripe papaya, peeled and seeded
- 1 cup pineapple chunks
- 1/2 cup coconut milk
- 1/2 cup Greek yogurt
- 1 tablespoon honey or maple syrup (optional)
- Ice cubes (optional)

Instructions:

1. Add all the ingredients to a blender.

2. Blend until the mixture is smooth and creamy.

3. If desired, add ice cubes and blend again for a refreshing chill.

4. Pour into a glass and enjoy the soothing tropical taste of this gut-soothing papaya and pineapple smoothie.

Gut-Healthy Chocolate Banana Smoothie

Ingredients:

- 1 ripe banana
- 2 tablespoons cocoa powder
- 1 tablespoon almond butter
- 1 cup almond milk
- 1 tablespoon honey or maple syrup (optional)
- Ice cubes (optional)

Instructions:

1. Place all the ingredients in a blender.
2. Blend until the mixture is velvety smooth.
3. If desired, add ice cubes and blend again for a frosty delight.

4. Pour into a glass and indulge in the rich and satisfying flavor of this gut-healthy chocolate banana smoothie.

Gut-Nourishing Matcha Green Tea Smoothie

Ingredients:

- 1 teaspoon matcha green tea powder
- 1 cup spinach
- 1/2 cup almond milk
- 1/2 cup Greek yogurt
- 1 tablespoon honey or maple syrup (optional)
- Ice cubes (optional)

Instructions:

1. Add all the ingredients to a blender.
2. Blend until the mixture is well incorporated and smooth.
3. If desired, add ice cubes and blend again for a chilled treat.

4. Pour into a glass and enjoy the earthy notes of this gut-nourishing matcha green tea smoothie.

Gut-Healing Turmeric and Ginger Smoothie

Ingredients:

- 1 cup pineapple chunks
- 1 small carrot, peeled and chopped
- 1/2 inch turmeric root, peeled
- 1/2 inch ginger root, peeled
- 1/2 cup coconut water
- 1/2 cup almond milk
- 1 tablespoon honey or maple syrup (optional)
- Ice cubes (optional)

Instructions:

1. Combine all the ingredients in a blender.
2. Blend until the mixture is smooth and creamy.
3. If desired, add ice cubes and blend again for a refreshing twist.

4. Pour into a glass and savor the zingy flavors of this gut-healing turmeric and ginger smoothie.

Gut-Friendly Avocado and Kale Smoothie

Ingredients:

- 1/2 ripe avocado
- 1 cup kale
- 1/2 green apple, cored and chopped
- 1/2 cup almond milk
- 1/2 cup coconut water
- 1 tablespoon lemon juice
- Ice cubes (optional)

Instructions:

1. Place all the ingredients in a blender.
2. Blend until the mixture is creamy and well blended.
3. If desired, add ice cubes and blend again for a chilled sensation.

4. Pour into a glass and enjoy the creamy and nutritious goodness of this gut-friendly avocado and kale smoothie.

Gut-Soothing Blueberry and Almond Butter Smoothie

Ingredients:

- 1 cup blueberries
- 1 tablespoon almond butter
- 1/2 cup Greek yogurt
- 1/2 cup almond milk
- 1 tablespoon honey or maple syrup (optional)
- Ice cubes (optional)

Instructions:

1. Add all the ingredients to a blender.
2. Blend until the mixture is smooth and luscious.
3. If desired, add ice cubes and blend again for a refreshing treat.

4. Pour into a glass and relish the delightful combination of blueberries and almond butter in this gut-soothing smoothie.

Gut-Healthy Watermelon and Mint Smoothie

Ingredients:

- 2 cups watermelon, seeded and cubed
- 1/4 cup fresh mint leaves
- 1/2 cup coconut water
- Juice of 1 lime
- Ice cubes (optional)

Instructions:

1. Combine all the ingredients in a blender.
2. Blend until the mixture is smooth and well blended.
3. If desired, add ice cubes and blend again for a cooling effect.
4. Pour into a glass and enjoy the refreshing and hydrating properties of this gut-healthy watermelon and mint smoothie.

Gut-Nourishing Peach and Coconut Smoothie

Ingredients:

- 1 ripe peach, pitted and sliced
- 1/2 cup coconut milk
- 1/2 cup Greek yogurt
- 1 tablespoon honey or maple syrup (optional)
- Ice cubes (optional)

Instructions:

1. Place all the ingredients in a blender.
2. Blend until the mixture is creamy and velvety.
3. If desired, add ice cubes and blend again for a chilled delight.
4. Pour into a glassand savor the sweet and tropical flavors of this gut-nourishing peach and coconut smoothie.

CONCLUSION

As we reach the end of this cookbook, I encourage you to continue prioritizing your gut health. Remember that small changes can make a big difference. Start by incorporating some of the recipes from this cookbook into your daily routine and observe how your body responds. Pay attention to how you feel after meals, any changes in digestion, and overall well-being.

Additionally, it is essential to remember that gut health is not solely dependent on diet. Lifestyle factors such as stress management, regular exercise, and adequate sleep also play a crucial role. Incorporating stress-reduction techniques like meditation, yoga, or engaging in activities that bring you joy can contribute to a healthier gut.

If you have any specific dietary concerns or conditions, I recommend consulting with a healthcare professional or a registered dietitian who specializes in gut health. They can provide personalized advice and guidance tailored to your unique needs.

Furthermore, as science continues to evolve, stay curious and up-to-date with the latest research in gut health. New discoveries are constantly being made, and it is exciting to witness the advancements in this field. Stay connected to reputable sources, attend workshops, and explore books and articles that delve deeper into gut health.

Lastly, I want to express my gratitude to you for embarking on this journey towards better gut health. By investing in your well-being, you are taking a proactive step toward a healthier and happier life. Remember that everyone's journey is unique, and progress may take time. Be patient and kind to yourself throughout the process.

I hope this cookbook has provided you with valuable insights, inspiration, and delicious recipes to support your gut health. May your gut thrive, and may you experience the numerous benefits that come with a healthy and balanced digestive system.